Contents

Contributors

Rob Butler
Consultant in Psychiatry of the Elderly, Mental Health, St Margaret's Hospital, Epping, Essex

Matthew Chester-Jones
Clinical Psychologist, Mental Health Unit, Princess Alexandra Hospital, Harlow, Essex

Stephen Davies
Honorary Senior Lecturer in Psychology, Royal Free and University College Medical School; Clinical Psychologist, Mental Health Unit, Princess Alexandra Hospital, Harlow, Essex

Angela Hassiotis
Senior Lecturer in Learning Disabilities, Royal Free and University College Medical School, Department of Psychiatry and Behavioural Sciences, London

Cornelius Katona
Professor of Psychiatry of the Elderly, Royal Free and University College Medical School, Department of Psychiatry and Behavioural Sciences, London

Gill Livingston
Reader in Mental Health of Older People, Royal Free and University College Medical School, Department of Psychiatry and Behavioural Sciences, London

Brice Pitt
Emeritus Professor of Old Age Psychiatry, Imperial College; Director, Hammersmith Memory Clinic, Hammersmith Hospital, London

Karen Shaw
Research Nurse, Parkinson's Disease Society Brain Research Centre, Institute of Neurology, London

Tim Stevens
Lecturer in Psychiatry of the Elderly, Royal Free and University College Medical School, Department of Psychiatry and Behavioural Sciences, London

Ajaya Upadhyaya
Consultant in Psychiatry of the Elderly, Mental Health Unit, Princess Alexandra Hospital, Harlow, Essex

Zuzana Walker
Senior Lecturer in Psychiatry of the Elderly, Royal Free and University College Medical School, Department of Psychiatry and Behavioural Sciences, London; Honorary Consultant, Mental Health, St. Margaret's Hospital, Epping, Essex

WT 230

The Memory Clinic Guide

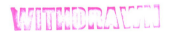

The Memory Clinic Guide

Edited by

Zuzana Walker
Senior Lecturer
Psychiatry of the Elderly
Royal Free and University College
Medical School, London

Rob Butler
Consultant in Psychiatry of the Elderly
Mental Health
St Margaret's Hospital, Epping, Essex

ealthcare Library
ospect Park Hospital
ney End Lane
ading RG30 4EJ
18 960 5012

MARTIN DUNITZ

© 2001 Martin Dunitz Ltd

First published in the United Kingdom in 2001 by
Martin Dunitz Ltd
The Livery House
7–9 Pratt Street
London NW1 0AE

Tel:	+44 (0)20 7482 2202
Fax:	+44 (0)20 7267 0159
E-mail:	info.dunitz@tandf.co.uk
Website:	http://www.dunitz.co.uk

All rights reserved. No part of this publication may be reproduced, stored in a retrieval
system, or transmitted, in any form or by any means, electronic, mechanical, photocopying,
recording or otherwise, without the prior permission of the publisher or in accordance with
the provisions of the Copyright, Designs and Patents Act 1988, or under the terms of any
licence permitting limited copying issued by the Copyright Licensing Agency, 90 Tottenham
Court Road, London W1P 0LP.

A CIP catalogue record for this book is available from the British Library

ISBN 1-84184-099-8

Distributed in the USA by
Fulfilment Center
Taylor & Francis
7625 Empire Drive, Florence, KY 41042, USA
Toll Free Tel.: +1 800 634 7064
E-mail: cserve@routledge_ny.com

Distributed in Canada by
Taylor & Francis
74 Rolark Drive
Scarborough, Ontario M1R 4G2, Canada
Toll Free Tel.: +1 877 226 2237
E-mail: tal_fran@istar.ca

Distributed in the rest of the world by
ITPS Limited
Cheriton House, North Way
Andover, Hampshire SP10 5BE, UK
Tel.: +44 (0)1264 332424
E-mail: reception@itps.co.uk

Printed and bound in Italy by Printer Trento S.r.l.

Preface

Over the past 20 years, memory clinics have evolved from an idea to an important part of many services for people with memory difficulties. The higher profile of the dementias, and Alzheimer's disease in particular, may mean that they have finally 'come of age' and those with dementia and their carers will receive the attention and resources they deserve. Hopefully, developments in genetics, imaging and therapeutics will continue to elucidate these illnesses and their treatments.

This short text is aimed at all health professionals who work in memory clinics or are interested in how memory clinics operate. We hope to have mentioned most aspects of setting up and running a memory clinic. We refer to longer texts for more details.

The contributors have worked at a number of different memory clinics, and all, at some stage, have worked at the Derwent Memory Clinic in Harlow and Epping, UK. Memory clinics have very different styles and approaches, often responding to local needs. We do not intend to lay down a blue print for the 'perfect' memory clinic but hope to stimulate professionals to provide even better memory clinics.

Zuzana Walker and Rob Butler

1

The history of memory clinics

Brice Pitt

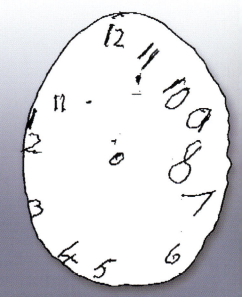

The first memory clinics

Memory clinics began in the USA in the early 1980s, largely through the enterprise of Thomas Crook and colleagues. These psychologists coined the term 'age-associated memory impairment' for forgetfulness and slowness to remember, which was presumed to arise from the dwindling powers of the ageing brain (Crook *et al.* 1986). An extensive battery of computerized memory tests, reflecting daily living activities such as shopping and driving, was used in a number of memory clinics in the USA and parts of Europe, sometimes being brought to communities in a bus (as with the *progetto memoria* in Italy). The first Crook-style memory clinic in the UK was established in Bradford.

Importance of research

At a time when concerns were growing about the ethics of obtaining 'informed' consent to participate in drug trials from people suffering from dementia, it seemed possible that people with age-associated memory impairment might provide an alternative group of subjects who were better able to give such consent. Indeed, the funding for memory clinics has often been met (in part, at least) by offering a free and comprehensive screening programme to older people, either referred by general practitioners or attracted by direct advertising, and then recruiting for drug trials those people who meet the criteria for dementia.

Memory clinics in the UK

Memory clinics started to appear in the UK later in the 1980s. A geriatrician, Norman Exton-Smith, set up the first such clinic. At his clinic at the Whittington Hospital, in London; an assessment included computerized testing and evoked potentials.

Geriatricians John Pathy and Tony Bayer in Cardiff, working with a psychologist, Charles Twining, described some success in finding reversible causes for apparent dementia among their first 100 cases. This suggested that the enterprise could be considerably cost-effective. A number of satellite memory clinics in Cardiff now bring the service ever closer to the community.

In the same year, a memory clinic at the Maudsley Hospital, in London, which was staffed by psychiatrists and a psychologist and which used computerized testing, was reported.

Probably the fourth memory clinic to be opened in the UK, in 1986, was the clinic at the Hammersmith Hospital, in London, with a psychiatrist, geriatrician, speech and language therapist and a psychologist.

At this stage it appeared that geriatrician-led clinics had an older clientele and a higher yield of demented patients than those developed by psychiatrists. Also, far more of those referred by general practitioners had dementia than those who referred themselves.

Populations using memory clinics

The growth of memory clinics in the UK was slow. Wright and Lindesay (1995) reported the activities of some 20 clinics – their staffing, assessments and research activity. On the whole it appeared that a memory clinic was regarded as something of a luxury for academic departments – an arena for dementia drug trials or simply a new name for the dementia outpatient clinic of an old-age psychiatry service. However, not everyone troubled by faulty memory would be seen willingly by such a service. Those under the age of 65 years would not be eligible, and where the problems arising from forgetfulness appeared mild or trivial, busy old age psychiatrists might not feel that their time would be well used in detailed appraisal. In a survey of London general practitioners before the opening of the Hammersmith Hospital Memory Clinic, the majority said that they would refer a patient complaining of a poor memory to a neurologist if 'young old', to a geriatrician if 'old old', to a psychiatrist if there were defective insight and behavioural problems, and perhaps to a psychologist if there were no insight or behavioural problems. Ninety-five per cent of those surveyed said that they would welcome a memory clinic (*Table 1.1*).

Table 1.1 People seen at memory clinics

✓ Usually patients aged over 50 years

✓ Patients with early dementia (with insight and without behavioural problems)

✓ Patients with milder cognitive impairment, without obvious pathology (e.g. age-associated memory impairment; memory impairment associated with substance abuse, epilepsy, cerebral vascular insufficiency, transient global amnesia, brain injury, unstable diabetes)

✓ Patients with dysphoric dysmnesia (related to depression, anxiety and stress)

✓ The 'worried well', who appear to have quite as good a memory as their peers but are fearful of becoming demented

Recent developments in the UK

The advent of the cholinesterase inhibitors – a rational approach to the treatment of Alzheimer's disease (though of transitory benefit and then only to some sufferers) – seems to have transformed the scene (see Chapter 5). There are now well over 100 memory clinics in the UK. Some have been set up with initial funding from drug companies. Others have been set up with a view to prescribing cholinesterase inhibitors in a well-regulated manner, with careful appraisal of their limitations and efficacy. This follows an unhappy 3 years of 'postcode prescribing' in the UK, when some Health Authorities have made the drugs readily available but others not at all (National Institute for Clinical Excellence, 2001). There is now a greater incentive to see patients who may have early dementia, and nurses and occupational therapists are playing a large part in new developments. What at first may have seemed a dilettante, super-specialized interest for academics and drug trials now looks like good clinical practice.

2

Setting up a memory clinic

Angela Hassiotis and Zuzana Walker

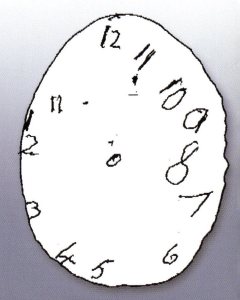

Models of memory clinics

There are many different models of memory clinics around the world. The set-up and the operating of a memory clinic depend mainly on the aims of the clinic. Some memory clinics are purely a research facility and some mainly provide a clinical service, but the majority have a dual potential. There is also a great variation in the extent of the clinical service. A memory clinic service can consist of a diagnostic assessment and a feedback session only, or it can provide on-going management. This chapter discusses the practicalities of setting up a memory clinic for which the main aim is to provide a clinical service while also encouraging training and research.

Funding

First, a decision has to be made about the funding of the clinic. In the past, memory clinics have frequently emerged from research projects that have been funded by commercial and charitable grants. More recently, an increasing number of memory clinics are set up and funded by health providers as they are becoming part of the standard care for the cognitively impaired elderly.

Setting and staffing

Memory clinics are usually, but not exclusively, linked to:

- old age psychiatry services;
- geriatric medicine services; or
- neurology services.

They are commonly based in outpatient departments or other health facilities, as they require a full complement of consulting rooms, including a waiting area, if possible with refreshment facilities.

Although the specialties involved can vary, depending or the local circumstances, the majority of memory clinics involve a multidisciplinary team. The minimum requirement is:

- a physician (e.g. a psychiatrist, a geriatrician, a neurologist); and
- another professional (e.g. a specialist nurse, a psychologist, a speech therapist, an occupational therapist).

To ensure the smooth running of a clinic, it is useful to have a co-ordinator of the clinic. This post can also have other clinical or administrative responsibilities within the memory clinic.

A memory clinic needs a room for performing a full physical examination, and it needs access to laboratory investigations and neuroimaging. Although in the UK, psychiatric departments often do not have a viewing box in examination rooms, it is advisable to have one in order to review computed tomography and magnetic resonance imaging scans. The basic facilities for a memory clinic are listed in *Table 2.1*.

Table 2.1 Basic facilities for a memory clinic

✓	Transport for patients and carers
✓	Two or more consultation rooms with a waiting area
✓	Examination couch
✓	Equipment for measuring blood pressure
✓	Equipment for neurological examination
✓	Viewing box for scans
✓	Equipment for neuropsychological testing including computers for computerized batteries of tests
✓	Database

Organization of the clinic

It is desirable that professionals have an opportunity to talk separately to informants and patients. This is best achieved by arranging the clinic so that while the patient sees one member of the team, the informant (a relative or carer) sees another member of the team.

Referrals

There are no fixed rules about the access route to the service and how referrals are made. This largely depends on local arrangements, but efforts should be made to identify and encourage referrals of those patients who would benefit most from a more in-depth, specialist evaluation. It is advisable to have a protocol that clearly spells out who is suitable to be seen in the memory clinic, and to have some form of screening of new referrals in place. It may be useful to suggest a cut-off score of, say, 20 out of 30 on the Mini Mental State Examination. For example, a 70-year-old patient who has Alzheimer's disease with severe behavioural disturbance and a Mini Mental State Examination score of 8 out of 30 would not be suitable, as he or she would not be able to understand and co-operate with the majority of schedules and tests.

Attendance

It is important that patients arrive for their appointments on time, since many professionals may be involved with the assessment of one patient during a given period. Therefore, delays can result in a considerable waste of clinical time.

A further problem is that of non-attendance. We have found it helpful to ask patients to confirm their attendance and, if possible, for a co-ordinator to remind them a few days before their appointment.

Assessment

The length of time of an assessment depends on the extent of the information to be gathered. The minimum time for an assessment would be approximately $1\frac{1}{2}$ hours, but if more extensive psychometric testing or formal psychiatric scales are carried out, an assessment could last several hours. In a survey of UK memory clinics, the mean time of an assessment was 3.1 hours (Wright and Lindesay 1995).

The ability of patients to co-operate with a lengthy assessment has to be taken into account, and in some cases an assessment might require more than one visit.

It is desirable, if tests are repeated, that testing takes place at the same time of the day, since patients can vary greatly during the day.

It is also helpful to have a regular multidisciplinary clinical meeting for case discussion and supervision; this meeting can also provide a focus for teaching and research activities.

Data collection and storage

Most services these days, even though they are not necessarily engaged in research activities, use a database to store and analyse the clinical information gathered. As with any other computerized records, the data protection rules must be observed and there should be a person dedicated to keeping the database up to date. It is also advisable to ask patients and carers in advance for permission to use computerized records, for purposes such as audit or research (see Chapter 7).

Memory clinics for people with learning disabilities

In recent years, the life expectancy of people with learning disabilities or mental retardation has greatly increased. As with the general population, longevity is associated with a higher risk and a higher prevalence of dementia. In particular, people with Down's syndrome are more susceptible to developing Alzheimer's disease in their 40s. Although some research into dementia in this group of patients has already been carried out, no specialized service for formal assessment of cognitive decline is available for this client group.

In November 1999, we established a memory clinic for people with learning disabilities jointly with our local memory clinic (the Derwent Memory Clinic at Harlow and Epping, UK). We have developed a protocol for the assessment and management of these patients that is based on the criteria of the American Association on Mental Retardation (*Table 2.2*) and we use a full battery of tests (see Chapter 4). The clinic is run once a month by two psychiatrists who specialize in learning disability and a psychologist who is linked to the mainstream memory clinic. Cases are discussed in joint meetings with the rest of the memory clinic team. This service has proved helpful for patients, carers and local services.

Table 2.2 American Association on Mental Retardation criteria for dementia in developmental disabilities

✓ Initial screening for dementia and periodic reviews
✓ All adults with Down's syndrome aged over 40 years and all others aged over 50 years
✓ Reversible causes of dementia
✓ Three-step course – recognize changes, conduct assessments and start medical and social care management

3

Medical assessment

Rob Butler

- History
- Mental state examination
- Physical examination
- Blood tests
- Imaging
- Further investigations

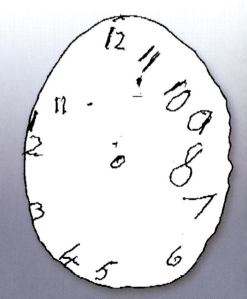

History

The history is the most important part of the medical assessment.

It is necessary to talk to an independent informant alone, if possible. Disparity and consistency between the subject's memory complaints and the informant's views are important.

The reason for referral should be established.

A careful attempt should be made to document when problems were first observed – early symptoms are helpful in making an accurate diagnosis.

The consequences, duration and progress of the memory problems should be recorded.

Questions should be asked about a wide range of cognitive domains as well as changes in role or personality.

It is important to record whether the patient drives, since patients with cognitive impairment need to stop driving until given permission from the licensing authorities. In addition, questions should be asked about:

- scholastic achievement;
- employment;
- marriage;
- children;
- retirement;
- medical and psychiatric history;
- current lifestyle, including alcohol, tobacco and benzodiazepine consumption;
- home and neighbours;
- activities and interests;
- worries and stresses.

It is useful to establish the patient's most taxing job so that their highest level of functioning can be compared to their present functioning.

Activities of daily living are listed in *Table 3.1*.

To get an accurate family history you need to draw a family tree and ask about each family member individually.

Table 3.1 Activities of daily living

✓ Personal hygiene and bathing
✓ Dressing
✓ Hobbies
✓ Meal preparation and eating
✓ Using household appliances
✓ Travelling
✓ Handling of correspondence
✓ Keeping appointments
✓ Handling finances
✓ Performance in employment

Mental state examination

Great care has to be taken not to confuse the following conditions with cognitive impairment:

- deafness;
- acute confusion;
- anger;
- irritability;
- anxiety;
- depression; and
- psychosis.

Particular attention needs to be paid to mood because depression is commonly associated with dementia, and treatment can improve the patient's functioning and the carer's quality of life.

Scales that cover a number of cognitive domains (e.g. memory, concentration, language, visuospatial abilities) complement cognitive testing (see Chapter 5). For a text on cognitive assessment, see Hodges (1994).

Delusions and hallucinations are common and need to be specifically asked for.

Behavioural difficulties include:

- restlessness;
- irritability;
- aggression;
- sexual disinhibition; and
- wandering.

It is important to assess the patient's own attitude to difficulties; patients with dementia often underestimate their level of cognitive impairment.

Physical examination

In addition to a standard physical examination, special emphasis should be given to certain aspects of the neurological examination:

- the fundi;
- the visual fields – defects can be easily missed in patients with dementia;
- primitive reflexes (grasp, pouting reflex) – their presence indicates loss of inhibition from the frontal cortex;
- focal signs – their presence suggests a diagnosis of cerebrovascular disease or a space-occupying lesion;
- tone in the limbs – increased tone is sometimes due to neuroleptic medication but it raises the possibility of dementia with Lewy bodies;
- bradykinesia and tremor – their presence in the early stages of a dementing illness also raises the possibility of dementia with Lewy bodies; and
- the gait – difficulty getting up or a shuffling gait suggests extrapyramidal disease.

Patients who persistently bump into objects on one side should be suspected of having a visual defect or neglect.

Assessment scales

There are a number of scales that are helpful for making a thorough assessment, arriving at a diagnosis, monitoring progress, and undertaking research. Achieving the correct balance between being thorough and not overtaxing your patients, their carers or the clinic staff is sometimes difficult. For each domain there is no 'perfect' scale because all scales suffer some limitations. Chapter 4 covers cognitive scales in some detail. *Table 3.2* lists other areas that may be tested with scales giving one example for each. For more details see McKeith (1999).

Table 3.2 Non-cognitive areas that may be tested with scales

Parameters measured	Example of a scale, with well-known abbreviations	Description
Global functioning	Clinical Global Impression of Change (CGIC)	Minimal guidelines, 7-point scale
Activities of daily living	Progressive Deterioration Scale (PDS)	27-point questionnaire completed by caregiver, takes about 15 minutes
Neuropsychiatric symptoms	The Neuropsychiatric Inventory with Caregiver Distress Scale (NPI-D)	Interview with carer covers 10 domains, takes about 10 minutes in the absence of symptoms
Depression	Cornell Scale for Depression in Dementia	Validated for people with dementia
Quality of life	Blau Quality of Life Scale (Blau QOL)	A generic quality of life scale covering many domains
Caregiver burden	Screen for Caregiver Burden	Self-report questionnaire, a useful screening instrument

Blood tests

There is no universal agreement on which blood tests make up a 'memory clinic screen'. However, as well as a few standard tests the choice of tests needs to be guided by the history and examination (*Table 3.3*). In the case of dementia, Chui and Zhang (1997) showed that the addition of laboratory tests changed the diagnosis in 9 per cent of patients and the management in 13 per cent.

Imaging

Magnetic resonance imaging (MRI) is the preferred scanning method for many memory clinics, but not all clinicians have access to MRI and it is more

Table 3.3 Blood tests for patients attending a memory clinic

Blood test	Indication
Full blood count	All patients
Erythrocyte sedimentation rate	All patients
Urea and electrolytes	All patients
Liver function tests	All patients
Calcium and phosphate	All patients
Thyroid function tests	All patients
Syphilis serology	All patients
Serum vitamin B_{12} and folate	All patients
Autoantibody screen	Younger patients and those with raised inflammatory markers or anaemia
C-reactive protein	Suspicion of an inflammatory process

expensive than computed tomography (CT). CT scans are also better tolerated by demented patients. The main aim of scanning is to exclude intracranial pathology such as:

- primary brain tumours;
- secondaries;
- chronic subdural haematomas;
- infarcts; and
- hydrocephalus.

Neuroimaging is essential for diagnosing vascular dementia according to some criteria. It is helpful in frontotemporal dementia, in which it shows preferential frontotemporal atrophy. Perfusion single photon emission tomography is particularly useful in the differential diagnosis of frontotemporal dementia, in which it shows a characteristic frontotemporal perfusion defect compared with a mainly temporoparietal hypoperfusion in Alzheimer's disease.

Further investigations

An electroencephalogram may assist in:

- distinguishing depression or delirium from dementia; and
- evaluating for suspected encephalitis, metabolic encephalopathy or seizures.

Nerve conduction studies are indicated in patients with evidence of muscle fasciculation.

Lumbar puncture for cerebrospinal fluid analysis is performed with an atypical progressing disease when central nervous system inflammation is suspected.

A tonsillar biopsy can confirm new variant Creutzfeldt–Jakob disease.

A brain biopsy may be performed in exceptional circumstances if a treatable cause of dementia is suspected (e.g. primary central nervous system vasculitis).

4

Psychometric assessment

Stephen Davies

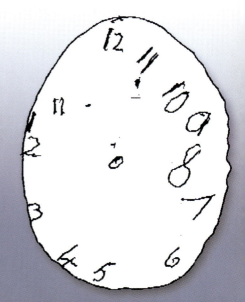

Background

A comprehensive assessment of memory problems requires three elements:

- a medical consultation;
- neuroimaging; and
- psychometric testing.

Psychometric test results add important information to the diagnostic and intervention processes, and they provide a statistical comparison of an individual's cognitive performance with a representative sample of similar people.

There are several texts (e.g. Berrios and Hodges, 2000) that provide detailed neuropsychological accounts of cognitive processes, particularly in the memory clinic's principal area of activity, the dementias.

Why do psychometric tests?

There are a number of reasons for doing psychometric tests (*Table 4.1*). As more resources become available for early intervention in dementia, the role of a basic psychometric profile becomes important for accessing entry to neuropsychological rehabilitation programmes and for comparison at follow-up.

With the advent of cholinesterase inhibitors, some countries now insist on psychometric test scores as an indicator for initiating and withdrawing treatment.

Table 4.1 Purposes of psychometric testing

✔ To determine the presence of cognitive deficits
✔ To measure the nature and scope of such deficits
✔ As a diagnostic aid
✔ As a treatment aid
✔ As a baseline for future assessments

Dignity and self-esteem may be affronted by test batteries, so administration is probably more appropriate in a memory clinic setting that is looking to provide an early identification service, rather than in a population in whom cognitive impairment has already been established.

Choice of psychometric tests

The Derwent Memory Clinic in the UK, in common with most memory clinics, uses a broad psychometric test battery as part of the initial memory clinic assessment (*Table 4.2*). Bucks and Loewenstein (1999) provide information on a number of psychometric test batteries that are used internationally.

Table 4.2 Derwent Memory Clinic psychometric test battery, with well-known abbreviations

✓ Mini Mental State Examination (MMSE)
✓ National Adult Reading Test (NART)
✓ Cambridge Cognitive Examination (CAMCOG)
✓ Logical Memory Test, Wechsler Memory Scale III
✓ Benton Controlled Oral Word Association Test (COWAT)
✓ Halstead Trail Making Test (TMT)
✓ British Picture Vocabulary Scales (BPVS)
✓ Coloured Progressive Matrices (CPM)
✓ CAMCOG-LD (unvalidated to date; adapted for use with people with learning disabilities)

It is important to consider the balance between breadth of assessment and the restraints that patient time and fatigue impose. Important factors for selecting a test battery are listed in *Table 4.3*.

The core elements of a psychometric test battery are listed in *Table 4.4*. Some or most elements of a test battery can now be offered on a computer. This can be a cost-effective, accurate, useful and viable option for many memory clinics. Wesners *et al.* (1999) provide a good summary of computerized test batteries.

Who administers psychometric tests?

Any health professional, with additional training, can administer a screening psychometric test battery. However, a psychology graduate with a background

Table 4.3 Factors in choosing a test battery

✓ Tests with ceiling settings (not too easy) and floor settings (not too hard) that are appropriate for the target population
✓ Tests with age-appropriate and culturally appropriate norms
✓ Tests with separate assessment of cognitive functions (e.g. memory, language)
✓ Tests with a risk–benefit analysis

Table 4.4 Core elements of a psychometric test battery

✓ Intelligence (premorbid and current)
✓ Memory (verbal and visual, recall and recognition)
✓ Language (production and comprehension)
✓ Executive functions (rule shifting and multiple concurrent element tasks)
✓ Perception (construction skills, spatial and object awareness)
✓ Laterality awareness

in psychometrics can offer special skills. It is important, if possible, that every memory clinic has access to a neuropsychologist who can:

- supervise the development and maintenance of the test battery;
- train and supervise relevant personnel; and
- provide specialist neuropsychological assessments and interventions.

How are psychometric tests carried out?

The way that a psychometric test battery is administered, and the person's reaction to it, may be as important as the quantitative results that it produces. The test environment should be maximally optimized and humanized.

If tests appear consistently too difficult or irrelevant to everyday cognitive skills, it may be difficult to convince an anxious and increasingly distressed patient to continue with a psychometric test battery. It is necessary to motivate people undergoing these tests while upholding their absolute right to dignified interaction and refusal to participate or to continue to participate. Non-completion should be thought of as the fault of the test battery, not of the person. Pursuit of psychometric test scores is unnecessary when reaction to the psychometric testing process can provide useful information.

Depression is the single largest confounder of psychometric test scores and should always be borne in mind when considering the presence of cognitive impairment.

When should psychometric testing be repeated?

There is a debate about how often to repeat psychometric testing. Psychometric test batteries without parallel forms (different versions of the same tests with varying but validated content) present problems because of learning effects that can confound results. There is a general consensus that repeat testing should not occur in less than 6 months. Some authors prefer a 1-year interval.

Special considerations

You may need to give special consideration for assessing some people at a memory clinic. People with severe sensory problems may need emphasis on an intact modality (e.g. drawing in the case of a hearing-impaired person) and the sensitive withdrawal of those tests that are not suited to their sensory status (e.g. long dictation passages).

People with physical disability may need to have special equipment or parts of the test battery omitted from their assessment.

People with learning disabilities are now forming a more significant proportion of memory clinic referrals as awareness about the possible differential vulnerability of certain groups of people with learning disabilities to dementia has been raised. This is a group of people that requires specialist psychometric assessment, and a number of developments to and adaptations of widely used psychometric instruments have been undertaken (see Chapter 2).

5 Medical interventions

Ajaya Upadhyaya

- Breaking the news
- Cholinesterase inhibitors
- Other possible cognitive enhancers
- Medications for associated conditions
- Genetic advice
- Support for carers

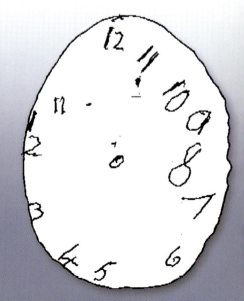

Breaking the news

In most memory clinics, the assessment session is followed by a feedback session to discuss the investigation results, the diagnosis and the future management with the patient and carers.

> Breaking the diagnosis of dementia needs to be done with tact and sensitivity and in an unhurried manner.
>
> Dementia is a catastrophic illness with devastating consequences.

Patients and carers often have questions about practical issues, including fitness to drive and the management of finances. The majority of patients and carers welcome a frank and open discussion, although in some cases carers express concern about the disclosure of the diagnosis to the patient. In these cases, it may be helpful to explain to the carers that most people do want to know their diagnosis and have the right to do so.

The blow of the diagnosis can be softened by the prospect of treatment, which, although not curative, can slow the progression of the disease. However, not all dementia sufferers are suitable for drug treatment. In contrast, virtually all patients and carers appreciate advice and information about practical and emotional help.

Cholinesterase inhibitors

Cholinesterase inhibitors are presently the most important group of medications for cognitive enhancement (for a review, see Mayeux and Sano, 1999). There are three drugs licensed for the treatment of Alzheimer's disease in the UK (Table 5.1):

- donepezil;
- rivastigmine; and
- galantamine.

Several randomized controlled trials have established that these medications lead to a modest but clinically important improvement in cognitive function, behavioural symptoms and activities of daily living in patients with mild to moderate Alzheimer's disease. Clinical experience suggests that these drugs may also benefit patients with other dementias, such as dementia with Lewy bodies.

Table 5.1 Cholinesterase inhibitors

Drug	Action	Half-life	Dose	Potential for drug interactions
Donepezil	Reversible inhibitor of acetylcholinesterase	70–80 hours	5–10 mg/day, in a single dose	Yes
Rivastigmine	Relatively selective pseudoirreversible inhibitor of acetyl-cholinesterase and butyrylcholinesterase	1–2 hours	6–12 mg/day, in two divided doses	Low
Galantamine	Reversible inhibitor of acetylcholinesterase and, to a negligible degree, of butyrylcholinesterase, with some nicotinic agonist activity	6 hours	16–24 mg/day, in two divided doses	Possible

Since higher doses of cholinesterase inhibitors appear to have the greatest therapeutic effect, but also the most adverse effects, the dose needs to be gradually titrated to improve tolerability and maximize the benefits. Common side effects of these drugs are listed in *Table 5.2*. Treatment can be continued indefinitely but the most common reasons for discontinuing therapy are side effects or lack of efficacy. In the UK, the National Institute for Clinical Excellence (2001) has suggested that cholinesterase inhibitors should be withdrawn, for a trial period, if the Mini Mental State Examination score falls below 12 out of 30.

Other possible cognitive enhancers

Gingko biloba is the best known non-medical agent. It has putative antioxidant, neurotropic and anti-inflammatory properties, and there is some evidence that it slightly improves cognitive functions in patients with Alzheimer's disease and vascular dementia. *Gingko biloba* is marketed as a health supplement and is available in health-food shops.

Table 5.2 Common side effects of cholinesterase inhibitors

✓	Nausea
✓	Vomiting
✓	Diarrhoea
✓	Abdominal pain
✓	Anorexia
✓	Insomnia

Controlled trials have shown vitamin E (alpha-tocopherol at a dose of 2000 IU), which limits free radical formation and promotes survival of cultured neurones exposed to beta-amyloid to improve proxy measures of function but not cognition in patients with Alzheimer's disease.

Selegiline has antioxidant properties and has been shown to be superior to placebo in delaying institutionalization or death.

Although inflammatory processes are implicated in Alzheimer's disease, diclofenac, an anti-inflammatory drug, has not been shown to produce benefits in a controlled trial.

Oestrogens may have some beneficial protective effect but more trials are needed.

Medication for associated conditions

Patients with dementia frequently suffer from depression and anxiety. Detection of an associated mood disorder and treatment with antidepressants can considerably improve a patient's functioning and quality of life. Several randomized controlled trials have shown that antidepressants may be effective for treating depression with dementia. However, the depression fluctuates and this is reflected in a high response rate to placebo.

An antidepressant, an antipsychotic or a mood stabilizer are sometimes indicated for treatment of associated behavioural symptoms, which are a source of significant distress to carers. Care must be taken to monitor carefully for side effects.

Genetic advice

The discovery of autosomal mutations in early-onset Alzheimer's disease and the association of apolipoprotein E_4 with late-onset disease have raised hopes for genetic testing to aid diagnosis and prediction. For example, in a patient with a family history of early-onset dementia suggestive of an autosomal dominant pattern, the presence of mutations in presenilin 1 and 2 or the apolipoprotein precursor protein gene would support the diagnosis of familial Alzheimer's disease.

However, in practice, genetic tests have limited usefulness. First, autosomal dominant mutations account for a small fraction of dementias. Second variable gene expression and incomplete penetrance limit the predictive value of mutations. Furthermore, these tests offer no benefit for sporadic cases of early-onset Alzheimer's disease or for late-onset Alzheimer's disease, the vast majority of which have no family history. Testing for apolipoprotein E_4 is not recommended for aiding diagnosis or predicting the development of Alzheimer's disease because the presence of apolipoprotein E_4 indicates increased risk but is not predictive of the disease. Predictive testing in asymptomatic members of families in which causative mutations have been discovered is problematic because of difficulties in interpreting the results. There are also important ethical considerations.

Therefore, genetic testing should usually be restricted to specialized centres. Careful screening, informed consent and counselling before and after the tests can then be offered.

An important aspect of caring for dementia sufferers is practical and emotional help to carers.

Support for carers

The vast majority of carers need information about practical issues to enable them to continue caring for as long as they wish to. This includes financial benefits (in the UK, Attendance Allowance) and domiciliary care. Voluntary services such as the Citizens Advice Bureaux and Age Concern are excellent resources of information and guidance in this area. The Alzheimer's Society is another good source of support for carers and they have local as well as a national network of centres. Most people need to be directed to local social services that arrange an appropriate care package after an assessment of needs for the patient and the carers.

Carers often need to be reminded of their own needs, which invariably includes some form of respite care. This can be provided through day care, a sitting-in service or relief admission. Some carers need more intensive therapy, including psychiatric intervention.

Longer-term care for patients is usually offered by local community mental health teams or general practitioners. As dementia progresses, supervised or residential accommodation may become necessary for the optimal welfare of the patient and the family.

6 Psychological interventions

Matthew Chester-Jones

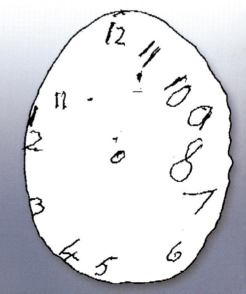

Challenges

There are particular challenges to providing rehabilitation for people with memory difficulties:

- since there is an impaired ability to learn and remember strategies, remediation often requires extensive training and support;
- dementing illnesses, by definition, are conditions of multiple impairments, so other impairments may limit strategy acquisition and use;
- impairment may be incorrectly considered global and progressive, and patients influenced by negative attitudes may be pessimistic about rehabilitation; and
- challenging behaviours associated with disease progression may interfere with rehabilitation.

Rehabilitation interventions

Rehabilitation interventions broadly divide into therapeutic approaches and cognitive strategies.

Therapeutic approaches

Therapeutic approaches generally aim to improve the well-being of patients, usually in later illness stages, and are useful in the day centre or residential setting (*Table 6.1*). No particular approach appears significantly more helpful than another, but they provide a rationale for carer–patient engagement, and they afford structure to aspects of the environment and daily routine.

Cognitive approaches

Cognitive approaches are usually offered in small group or individual interventions. Post-diagnosis supportive groups provide opportunities for both patients and carers to meet and share with others in the same situation, addressing the isolation and taboo associated with mental impairment.

Later, interventions are usefully directed towards carers. Apart from needing support, carers can learn the rehabilitation strategies available, decide which will improve their quality of life, and apply them individually at home.

Conceptualization of memory

Memory can be conceptualized according to psychological processes or temporal (time) domains. Successful learning entails attending to material at hand, then registering it meaningfully or in detail. Successful memory entails retaining the material integrally, then retrieving it appropriately in recognition or recall. There is retrograde memory for prior learning and experience; and anterograde memory

Table 6.1 Therapeutic approaches and brief descriptions

Therapeutic approach	Brief description
Stimulation or activity programmes	Includes activities such as music and dance to increase the number of pleasant activities to improve the mood of patients and carers
Reality orientation	Provides accurate information to orientate the person to his or her surroundings
Reminiscence	Encourages people to talk about the past in order to bring past experiences into consciousness
Life review	Preserved longer term memories can be used to make sense of one's life
Validation approaches	Seek to restore self-worth and decrease stress by validating emotional ties to the past

for new or recently acquired learning. Prospectively, there is working memory for immediate tasks and short-term goals; and prospective memory for events in the further future.

Thorough assessment of memory functioning is essential for successful rehabilitation. Identifying strengths in memory processes, and temporal domains, is a valuable goal for rehabilitation (for a review, see Butters *et al.* 1998).

Strategies for registration and retention

A useful general strategy is to reduce cognitive load at registration by:

- breaking material down into smaller chunks of information (e.g. telephone number 83369472 could become 833 694 72); or
- providing shorter steps in a sequence (e.g. ironing a shirt becomes 'collars, cuffs, sides, sleeves').

Another strategy is to reduce distraction by offering a quiet, uncluttered, environment.

Some patients may learn to use mnemonic or associative strategies. These include the loci method (e.g. imagining a series of targets in each of the rooms at home) or associating a name with a face by imagining a visual connection (e.g. Dr Brown, who has brown hair).

Other patients may benefit from verbal mediation. This includes verbally 'stamping' an activity (e.g. saying out loud, 'I am placing my diary on the sideboard') or rehearsing a task (e.g. silently repeating, 'I am going upstairs to fetch my glasses').

Less able patients may be helped to learn or regain skills by supported learning techniques such as:

- backward chaining;
- errorless learning;
- vanishing cues; and
- spaced retrieval.

For example, in spaced retrieval, the patient practises an activity at slowly increasing intervals – the newly learned information is first repeated 5 minutes after learning, then 10 minutes after this, then 15 minutes later and so on.

Strategies for retrieval

One general strategy is to reduce anxiety associated with retrieval. Patients can use relaxation techniques such as muscular relaxation or positive visualization to aid recall.

Another strategy is to increase structure in the environment by labelling drawers and doors at home or by initiating a regular daily routine.

Some able patients may use self-cuing techniques such as mental retracing (e.g. of the activities that preceded the loss of a particular item) or context recreation (e.g. of the circumstances of an important conversation).

Many patients require external aides to memory (*Table 6.2*).

Suggested cognitive rehabilitation group

Three or four patients and their main carer may be invited to attend for six weekly, one-hour sessions:

- Build on prior knowledge by introducing the temporal domains as past (retrograde), present (working) and future (prospective) memory.
- Discuss strategies already used by the group (e.g. common rhyming mnemonics, diaries, notebooks) and present structured alternatives.
- Introduce the 'memory folder', comprising three sections:

- in a 'past memory' section, patients build up a reference library of life events, important people and personal data in an individual form (e.g. stories, lists, photographs);
- 'present memory' comprises a day-to-view diary page of scheduled routine, to-do lists and instructions related to times of the day – this page can be annotated by the patient at the end of the day and added to the 'past memory' section as a log of events or experiences;
- 'future memory' contains a few week-to-view diary pages marked with planned activities, and a one-page list of anniversaries and seasonal and long-term commitments.

- Memory folders are easily word-processed and adapted to individual patient needs. As each section is presented, patients are invited to try it out as that week's homework.
- Introduce general strategies, including relaxation techniques and changes to environment and routine (for further suggestions, see Sohlberg and Mateer 1989).

Table 6.2 External aides to memory

Aide	Examples
Written reminders for on-going tasks	Shopping lists, mealtime instructions
Timers or alarms to help to cue goals	Alarm to tell the patient when to turn off the oven or take a medicine
A daily planner	Appointment book or calendar (useful for remote activity and events)
Specialist watches	Pagers and mobile phones may provide an alarm for action (e.g. time to take a medicine) supported by a verbal prompt (e.g. which medicine to take)

7 Research

Cornelius Katona and Gill Livingston

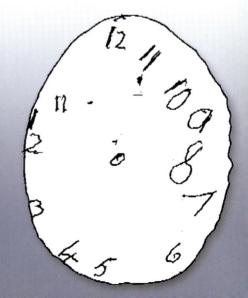

Obtaining consent

Particular care is required to ensure that people with possible or definite cognitive impairment are given the opportunity to make as informed a decision as possible about whether to participate in research.

Many research ethics committees provide some local guidelines as to how best to achieve this. Potential participants should have the proposed procedures explained to them with due attention to problems with hearing and understanding. They should also be given an information sheet (expressed as simply as possible and in large print) that they can discuss at leisure with a carer, relative or friend who is unconnected with the research, or with their general practitioner. *Table 7.1* lists important points that should be explained as clearly as possible.

Although no one can give consent on behalf of an adult, it is good practice to involve and inform carers. Research may in some circumstances be carried out ethically with patients who lack the competence to give informed consent but who agree to the research. This is termed 'assent'; family carers should also be asked for permission in these circumstances.

Clinical databases

Clinical databases fall within the provisions of the Data Protection Act (1998). The Act addresses the responsibilities of researchers (or other 'data controllers') who are in possession of data that relate to a living person who could be identified either directly or with the use of additional information in the hands of the data controller. The data subject is entitled to know a number of facts (*Table 7.2*).

Table 7.1 Important points to explain when obtaining consent

✓ The nature and purpose of the research
✓ The participant's proposed contribution
✓ That clinical care will not be affected by participation or otherwise in the research
✓ That participants can withdraw consent at any time and do not need to give a reason

Table 7.2 Information that a database subject has the right to know

✓ What is being processed
✓ The purpose for which it is being processed
✓ The recipient(s) to whom it is being or might be disclosed
✓ An intelligible explanation of any codes used

This means that formal consent (see above) needs to be sought from each memory clinic attender (or carer) to use information collected on a database for research purposes, and an explanation given of the specific use or uses to which such data will be put. Codes of Practice have not been developed, although the Information Commissioner plans to encourage them. It is unclear how this might affect datasets already collected or what the implications are of collecting data from cognitively impaired memory clinic attenders who can assent to but not give informed consent.

Potential areas of research

Memory clinics provide a wealth of research opportunities. We have reviewed the literature (using Medline and Embase 1994–2001, with the search terms 'memory clinic' and 'research'); the thematic summary below is based on this review and our own research experience.

Frequency of dementia subtypes

Memory clinics provide a good setting (albeit not a representative one) for studies examining the frequency of dementia subtypes. Swanwick et al. (1998) reported on a series of 200 consecutive memory clinic attenders and found that two-thirds fulfilled criteria for probable or possible Alzheimer's disease and other primary degenerative dementias; only 9 per cent had vascular dementias, with the remainder having mixed dementias.

A larger (n=400) and more recent study by Hogh et al. (1999) found that only 46 per cent had dementia; 19 per cent had other cognitive deficits. Potentially reversible conditions were found in 26 per cent. This sample was relatively young (mean age 64 years) and the clinic was neurology-led, rather than psychiatry-led.

Farina et al. (1999) reviewed 513 memory clinic attenders (mean age 69 years) and found that 71 per cent had dementia. Of particular note in their study was the subgroup (7 per cent) that had potentially reversible conditions. Half of this group had a complete reversal of cognitive decline after appropriate treatment, and a further one fifth had partial cognitive improvement.

Instruments for diagnosis

A further approach is to evaluate the usefulness of instruments in making a diagnosis. Coen *et al.* (1994) validated a new diagnostic instrument, the DAT inventory, against clinical criteria and found it to have good specificity (95 per cent) and satisfactory sensitivity (71 per cent). The DAT worked least well in very mild and atypical dementia, and best in mild-to-moderate dementia.

More recently, McKinnon and Mulligan (1998) examined the use of the Mini Mental State Examination, the short form of the IQ Code and a combination of the two for diagnosis. They demonstrated that using the instruments together resulted in a more accurate diagnosis than using either of them separately.

Neuropsychological profiles

Reid *et al.* (1996) found that Alzheimer's disease patients with a younger age of onset had more attentional impairment, more impairment of working memory and more apraxia than patients with late-onset disease. This suggests greater disruption of cortical pathways to the frontal lobes in patients with early-onset disease.

Walker *et al.* (1997) compared performance of people with Alzheimer's disease and dementia with Lewy bodies (matched for global dementia severity) on CAMCOG subscales and found that dementia with Lewy bodies was associated with relative preservation of recall but more impairment in visuospatial praxis.

Natural history

Swannick *et al.* (1998) found that the annual rate of change in people with Alzheimer's disease was highly variable, with age, duration and previous rate of decline all failing to predict the future annual rate of cognitive decline.

Visser *et al.* (2000) reported a prevalence of significant depression of 60 per cent in people with mild memory impairment. Within the depressed group, those who developed Alzheimer's disease 3–5 years later were older and had poorer cognitive performance at baseline.

It is likely that in future, as memory clinics take on a clinical role in monitoring new and established treatments for Alzheimer's disease and other dementias, naturalistic studies of treatment response will become an important focus for memory clinic research.

Neuroimaging

Many memory clinic patients have neuroimaging as part of their clinical work-up. Lavenu *et al.* (1997) examined the diagnostic value of the combination of medial temporal lobe atrophy on computed tomography and decreased temporoparietal uptake on single photon emission tomography. They found that the resultant index was specific but not sensitive for Alzheimer's disease.

Imaging studies in a memory clinic setting do not have to be restricted to referred patients. O'Brien *et al.* (1997) investigated the neuroradiological correlates of the rate of cognitive decline; they found that hippocampal atrophy (but not periventricular or deep white matter lesions) were associated with age-related cognitive decline in non-demented spouses of memory clinic attenders.

Carers

More generally, carer-focused research within memory clinics has turned out to be very fruitful. Coen *et al.* (1997) investigated predictors of carer burden in Alzheimer's disease and found that it was related mainly to lack of social support and increased patient behavioural problems but not to cognitive or functional status.

In a subsequent study (Coen *et al.* 1999), the same group evaluated the effect of a dementia carer education programme on carer quality of life, burden and well-being in a before–after design in a memory clinic setting. This programme increased carer knowledge but despite high carer satisfaction had no other effect.

In a similar pilot randomized controlled trial, Logiudice *et al.* (1999) compared memory clinic attendance with usual treatment. No significant effects on carer psychological morbidity, burden or knowledge of dementia were found, but there was a significant improvement in health-related quality of life.

Obtaining funding for research

Sadly there is no 'magic recipe' for success in obtaining funding. Many small projects can, however, be carried out within an established service with little or no additional funding. Clinically, to work well, a memory clinic needs to be adequately resourced. A well-functioning memory clinic attracts personnel seeking both clinical training and research experience (particularly psychiatrists and psychologists). Larger projects will of course require funding (in the UK, usually from NHS Research and Development or from the major research charities). Several factors associated with a greater likelihood of obtaining such funding are listed in *Table 7.3*.

Table 7.3 Factors associated with a greater likelihood of obtaining funding

✓ Choosing a funding body with an appropriate focus

✓ Demonstrating the clinical viability and 'through-put' of the memory clinic

✓ Carrying out small pilot projects exploring hypotheses and demonstrating the feasibility of the protocol

✓ Writing a hypothesis-driven protocol with clear justification of the sample size

8 Ending it well

Karen Shaw and Tim Stevens

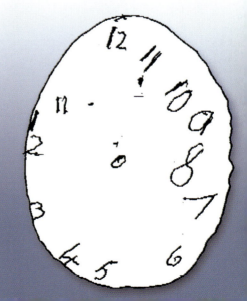

The place of post-mortems

The Renaissance idea that *mortui vivos docent* – 'the dead teach the living' – has become less fashionable in recent decades, and post-mortem rates have declined, possibly as diagnostic overconfidence has increased. Nonetheless, the definitive diagnosis of dementia remains histopathological, and histopathological examination must be assessed at post-mortem examination since antemortem brain biopsy is rarely justified. The obtaining of brains for post-mortem study, or 'brain donation', is an important part of a modern memory clinic.

Benefits

The benefits of a post-mortem are well recognized. For clinicians, these include the confirmation, clarification or refutation of antemortem diagnoses, allowing clinical practice to be improved (*Table 8.1*). Detailed psychiatric history and neuropsychological assessments of cognitive performance can be valuable when related to post-mortem findings.

For families of deceased patients, benefits include the comfort of certainty of diagnosis (*Table 8.2*).

Post-mortem examinations as part of diagnosis and management

Assessment in the memory clinic is usually offered to patients in the early stages of cognitive impairment. It may seem insensitive to ask the patient and his or her relatives to consider inevitable deterioration and death when a diagnosis has just been made. However, evidence suggests that many patients, aware of the prospect

Table 8.1 Benefits of brain donation for clinicians

✓ Confirmation, clarification and correction of antemortem diagnosis
✓ Evaluation of diagnostic tests
✓ Evaluation of new treatments
✓ Discovery and definition of new diseases
✓ Contribution to medical research and enhancement of research opportunities
✓ Reassurance of family members
✓ Opportunity for monitoring and documenting quality of care

Table 8.2 Benefits of brain donation for families

✓	Comfort from knowing cause of death
✓	Reassurance that all care was given
✓	'Good' coming from sadness and suffering, helping to alleviate guilt
✓	Discovery of hereditary disease
✓	Advancement of medical knowledge

of diminishing skills, wish to make plans, including the preparation of a will, advance directives about resuscitation, and application for enduring power of attorney. These measures may account for the finding that fear of death declines with age. During post-diagnostic counselling, the clinician may discuss the importance of brain donation for confirmation of the diagnosis and for research purposes.

Brain banks

Since the 1970s, so-called 'brain banks' have been set up throughout Europe to collect large numbers of brains from people with particular diseases. Recruitment of patients or control donors (a spouse may also be asked to donate his or her brain, as he or she will usually match well in areas of age, nutrition and social status) is a delicate task. Each patient should be approached with sensitivity, tact and empathy, and the donation request should be stated simply, directly and non-forcefully. Euphemistic phrases such as 'giving some of your brain tissue when the time comes' are not (in the authors' experience) helpful and tend to betray the clinician's own uneasiness about making the request.

Asking for consent

The discussion of post-mortem examination may provide an opportunity for the patient and his or her relatives to express a range of emotions and behaviours – from denial, anger, fear and refusal to consent, and from evasiveness to acceptance or positive willingness (*Table 8.3*). The clinician should anticipate sadness and grief and be prepared to offer appropriate bereavement counselling. In a sense, the raising of the practical issue of post-mortem brain donation can pave the way for acceptance by the patient and carer of the patient's inevitable death. Discussion should be encouraged within a family and time given to reach a decision.

Table 8.3 Basic principles for requesting and obtaining permission for post-mortem examination and for providing feedback about results

✓	Legal, ethical and administrative protocols should be in place from the outset
✓	Patients and relatives should be approached for consent early in the course of the illness and preferably shortly after diagnosis has been made
✓	Consent is more likely to be obtained if patients agree than if relatives are asked to provide consent on their behalf
✓	Both personal benefits and benefits to future generations should be stressed
✓	Refusal to consent may be based on inadequate information about the procedure, which should be remedied
✓	Prompt disclosure of post-mortem results should be offered and may be therapeutic for the relative

When the reasons for donation are understood, most people are willing to give consent. Rates of 75–85 per cent have been reported in obtaining consent for brain donation, with higher rates being obtained in patients and controls who were directly approached than in cases in which relatives were asked to provide consent on behalf of the sufferer. The oldest old have been found to be more likely to consent than the younger old.

Attitudes to brain donation

There is much literature on attitudes to post-mortem, and commonly expressed concerns by relatives are that their loved one has 'suffered enough', that there may be delays in funeral arrangements, and that disfigurement will result. Often carers of patients with dementia feel the person they knew is no longer there, and are consequently not opposed to donation. The opportunity to contribute towards medical research and help others in the future may enable relatives and patients to salvage some meaning from an otherwise hopeless situation.

However, not all patients and relatives have a positive view of brain donation. Feelings of fear and prejudice may be expressed, although a lack of understanding about the request can be overcome by clear information and explanation. Relatives may decline to provide consent if the patient has expressed negative attitudes toward post-mortem in the past, and in such cases the clinician must accept and respect this, and post-mortem will remain unobtainable.

Protocols

Clear legal, ethical and administrative protocols must be in place before any attempts are made to recruit patients or controls. This is of particular importance in the light of recent public concerns about the use of organs for research. The legal position as to the authority from which consent for post-mortem should be obtained is unclear (Medical Protection Society 1988), which further highlights the need for donation to be discussed early.

Families often eagerly await post-mortem feedback, and communicating the results without delay must be an integral part of the brain donation programme. Clinicians who conduct post-mortem discussion meetings frequently report that these help the bereaved to cope with their loss and grief, often bringing the matter to closure.

After death

Finally, the relatives should not be forgotten once the patient has died. Despite the best preparation, the loss of a loved one almost always has an emotional impact, and it is not uncommon for close carers to experience emotions that they may regard as shameful, such as relief. There is also the disorientation that accompanies the sudden changing of roles – the relative may suddenly find himself or herself with little to do. A discussion of the grieving process may be helpful, and the relatives should be encouraged to express even 'unacceptable' emotions and be reassured that these are common and normal.

References

Berrios G, Hodges J (2000) *Memory disorders in psychiatric practice.* Cambridge University Press, Cambridge.

Bucks RS, Lowenstein DA (1999) Neuropsychological assessment. In: Wilcock GS, Bucks RS, Rockwood K, eds. *Diagnosis and management of dementia: a manual for memory teams.* Oxford University Press, Oxford.

Butters MA, Soety EM, Glisky EL (1998) Memory rehabilitation. In: Snyder PJ, Nussbaum ND, eds. *Clinical neuropsychology: a pocket handbook for assessment.* American Psychiatric Association, Washington, DC.

Chui HC, Zhang Q (1997) Evaluation of dementia: a systematic study of the usefulness of the American Academy of Neurology's practice parameters. *Neurology* 49:925–35.

Coen RF, O'Boyle CA, Coakley D, *et al.* (1999) Dementia carer education and patient behaviour disturbance. *Int J Geriatr Psychiatry* 4:302–6.

Coen RF, Swanwick GR, O'Boyle CA, *et al.* (1997) Behaviour disturbance and other predictors of carer burden in Alzheimer's disease. *Int J Geriatr Psychiatry* 12:331–6.

Coen RF, O'Mahoney D, Bruce I, *et al.* (1994) Differential diagnosis of dementia: a prospective evaluation of the DAT Inventory. *J Am Geriatr Soc* 42:16–20.

Crook T, Bartus R, Ferris S, *et al.* (1986) Age-associated memory impairment: proposed diagnostic criteria and measure of clinical change. Report of a National Institute for Mental Health working group. *Dev Neuropsychol* 2:261–76.

Data Protection Act (1998) Crown Copyright.

Farina E, Pomati S, Mariani C (1999) Observations on dementias with possibly reversible symptoms. *Aging (Milano)* 11:323–8.

Hodges JR (1994) *Cognitive assessment for clinicians.* Oxford University Press, Oxford.

Hogh P, Waldemar G, Knudsen GM, *et al.* (1999) A multidisciplinary memory clinic in a neurological setting: diagnostic evaluation of 400 consecutive patients. *Eur J Neurol* 6:279–88.

Lavenu I, Pasquier F, Lebert F, *et al.* (1997) Association between medial temporal lobe atrophy on CT and parietotemporal uptake decrease on SPECT in Alzheimer's disease. *J Neurol Neurosurg Psychiatry* 63:441–5.

Logiudice D, Waltrowicz W, Brown K, *et al.* (1999) Do memory clinics improve the quality of life of carers? A randomized pilot trial. *Int J Geriatr Psychiatry* 14:626–32.

Mackinnon A, Mulligan R (1998) Combining cognitive testing and informant report to increase accuracy in screening for dementia. *Am J Psychiatry* **155**:1529–35.

Mayeux R, Sano M (1999) Treatment of Alzheimer's disease. *N Engl J Med* **341**:1670–9.

McKeith IG (1999) *Outcome measures in Alzheimer's disease.* Martin Dunitz, London.

Medical Protection Society (1988) *Consent, confidentiality, disclosure of medical records.* The Medical Protection Society, London.

National Institute for Clinical Excellence (2001) *Review for cholinesterase inhibitors.* National Institute for Clinical Excellence, London.

O'Brien JT, Desmond P, Ames D, *et al.* (1997) Magnetic resonance imaging correlates of memory impairment in the healthy elderly: association with medial temporal lobe atrophy but not white matter lesions. *Int J Geriatr Psychiatry* **12**:369–74.

Reid W, Broe G, Creasey H, *et al.* (1996) Age at onset and pattern of neuropsychological impairment in mild early-stage Alzheimer disease. A study of a community-based population. *Arch Neurol* **53**:1056–61.

Sohlberg MM, Mateer CA (1989) Training use of compensatory memory books: a three stage behavioural approach. *J Clin Exp Neuropsychol* **11**:871–91.

Swanwick GR, Coen RF, Coakley D, *et al.* (1998) Assessment of progression and prognosis in 'possible' and 'probable' Alzheimer's disease. *Int J Geriatr Psychiatry* **13**:331–5.

Visser PJ, Verhey FR, Ponds RW, *et al.* (2000) Distinction between preclinical Alzheimer's disease and depression. *J Am Geriatr Soc* **48**:479–84.

Walker Z, Allen RL, Shergill S, *et al.* (1997) Neuropsychological performance in Lewy body dementia and Alzheimer's disease. *Br J Psychiatry* **170**:156–8.

Wesnes KA, Hildebrand K, Mohr E (1999) Computerized cognitive assessment. In: Wilcock GK, Bucks RS, Rockwood K, eds. *Diagnosis and management of dementia: a manual for memory disorders teams.* Oxford University Press, Oxford.

Wright N, Lindesay J (1995) A survey of memory clinics in the British Isles. *Int J Geriatr Psychiatry* **10**:379–85.

Index

Healthcare Library
Prospect Park Hospital
Honey End Lane
Reading RG30 4EJ
0118 960 5012